A Review of Literature on Gastric Acidity

BY

Hafsa Tahir

PREFACE

Gastric acidity is a common complain these days. Almost 60 million people suffer from gastric acidity once in a month. Many people confuse it with angina pectoris. To know the root cause, complete understanding of human gut is important. In this book, I have tried to explain the reasons behind gastric acidity along with precautions and treatment.

Author: Hafsa Tahir

CONTENTS

Introduction.

Nowadays each fifth person suffers from stomach acidity – an imbalance between the stomach and proximal intestine structure and ensuring their safety protective mechanisms. The stomach usually secretes acid which helps to break down the food, but its excess ion leads to acidity (Stomach acidity symptoms, 2008, www.home-remedies-for-you.com).

The human digestive system is a complex and many sectioned biological mechanism designed to break down foods into small, easily absorbable particles and to eliminate the unusable remains.

The process of digestion begins in the mouth, at the top end of the 30 foot long alimentary canal. It continues down through the esophagus, stomach, small and large intestines, ending finally at the rectum where wastes from the digestive action are voided through the anal canal. The movement of food from the mouth to the rectum can take up to two to three days or more, depending on the efficiency and vitality of the organs processing it

In the process of digestion, food remnants are chemically transformed: carbohydrates are turned into small sugar molecules, protein into small peptides and amino acids, and fat into fatty acids and glycerol. These substances are absorbed into the cells lining the intestine, processed again, and transferred into the blood and lymphatic system for transport. They are then used as building blocks and energy-producing fuel for the entire body (Minocha, A etal, 2003).

1

The mouth

The moment we take a bite of food, salivary glands in the mouth secrete enzymes that break down complex sugars and starches into simple sugars. As the food literally starts to melt in the mouth, teeth chop and grind it even more, until the food forms a coarse bolus (ball) that is soft and pulpy enough to pass easily down the esophagus. While some of this food may be gulped, depending on chewing habits, a majority of it reaches the esophagus already well smoothed (Minocha, A etal, 2003).

The esophagus

The tongue and the swallowing muscles in the throat push the bolus of the food into the esophagus, a tube of muscle that is about 25 centimeter long. It starts at the bottom of the throat and ends at the stomach. The lower end of the esophagus is capped with the ring of muscle known as the lower esophageal sphincter. The ring opens when it senses pressure from the food, then closes once the food has passed through. As the bolus of food makes its way down to the esophagus, the esophagus contract rhythmically, moving the food quickly along and into the stomach (Minocha, A etal, 2003).

The stomach

The stomach is a segment of the gastrointestinal tract that participates in the digestion of food and other important philological responses to food. It is a muscular sac linking the esophagus and the first portion of the small intestine, known as the duodenum. Anatomically, it lies just below the diaphragm in the abdominal cavity. The primary functions of stomach are to begin the process of digestion and to serve as a reservoir for ingested food so that it can be delivered at a controlled rate to the segments of the intestine. This results in an optimal rate of digestion and absorption of ingested nutrients, so that the capacity of the small intestine for these processes is not overwhelmed.

The stomach is not required for normal digestion and absorption of nutrients to occur, but its dysfunction can result in several disease states (Minocha, A etal, 2003).

As the stomach fills up, it rhythmically relaxes and contracts, mixing the food, breaking it down into 1-2 millimeter particles and saturating it with gastric fluids. After two, three or more hours, of this intense churning, the food is finally broken down into a blended mixture known as chyme. A ring of muscle in the stomach known as the pyloric sphincter then open on an as-needed basis, accepting these thick liquid and sending portions of it into the small intestine (Minocha, A etal, 2003).

The small intestine

Once in small intestine, the chyme continues its journey its journey through the alimentary canal helped along by peristaltic action produced by muscle contractions. Further enzymatic break down takes place now, assisted by secretions from pancreas and from fat digesting bile sent to it by gallbladder and liver. The first part, a short, curved section of the intestines known as the duodenum, converts the aggravations of the fats, proteins and carbohydrates.

Eventually, substances in the intestines decompose to the point where they are molecularly small enough to absorb into the intestinal cells and be reprocessed for eventual transport by the blood and lymphatic system. These absorbed nutrients are then used by the body as building blocks and fuel to sustain the life of the organism.

Meanwhile, all undigested left overs of the food pass into the large intestine for final processing and absorption (Minocha, A etal, 2003).

The large intestine or colon

By the time food residues reach large intestine, the work of digestion and absorption is almost, but not quite, complete. It is now the job of the beneficial bacteria that line the colon to feed on these waste materials and convert some of them to useful nutrients for absorption (Minocha, A etal, 2003).

First, wastes in the colon are moved by peristalsis upward through a section known as the ascending colon. Then, they are passed horizontally across the transverse colon. Next, they move downward into the descending colon. Finally, as they near the end of the alimentary canal, they take a sharp turn along the sigmoid flexure and pass on into the rectum for disposal.

While moving through these various sections of the large intestine, the friendly flora that make their home along the colon wall, besides converting waste matter into feces, produce enzymes that perform the last bit of digestion, breaking down the stubborn particles of fiber and vegetable matter. All this time, the colon continues to absorb water and electrolytes. Finally, the long and remarkable task of digestion and absorption complete, the remaining indigestible residues are passed through the rectum and out in the form of feces (Minocha, A etal, 2003).

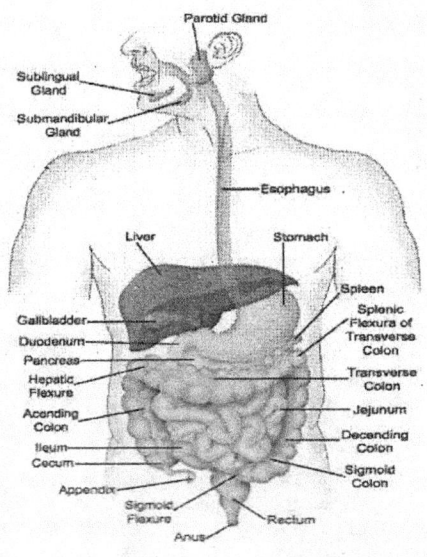

(2010, www.eatwellgetwell.files.wordpress.com)

ACIDITY

Acids are normally secreted by the stomach to facilitate the digestive process and help break down food. High levels of these stomach acids can however cause the condition called acidity (Sherwood, L.,2010).

Acid reflux is a chronic condition where acid flows up from the stomach into the esophagus causing acid indigestion or heartburn (Kate Gilbert, U., 2001).

The stomach secrets a number of characteristics products from cells that line its interior. Perhaps the best known of these is hydrochloric acid, secreted by so-called parietal cells located in glands that drain into the central portion of the stomach. Gastric acid is secreted in response to cues that a meal is about to, or has entered the stomach. The acidity begins the process of breaking down the large molecules present in a meal. The acid is highly toxic to the ingested bacteria and thus serves as a host defense mechanism (Stomach acidity, 2007, www.stomachacidity.com).

Gastric acid is a secretion produced in the stomach. It is one of the main solutions secreted, together with several enzymes and intrinsic factors. Chemically it is an acid solution with a pH of 1 to 2 in the stomach lumen, consisting mainly of hydrochloric acid (HCl) (around 0.5%, or 5000 parts per million), and large quantities of potassium chloride (KCl) and sodium chloride (NaCl) (Guyton, A. C etal, 2006).

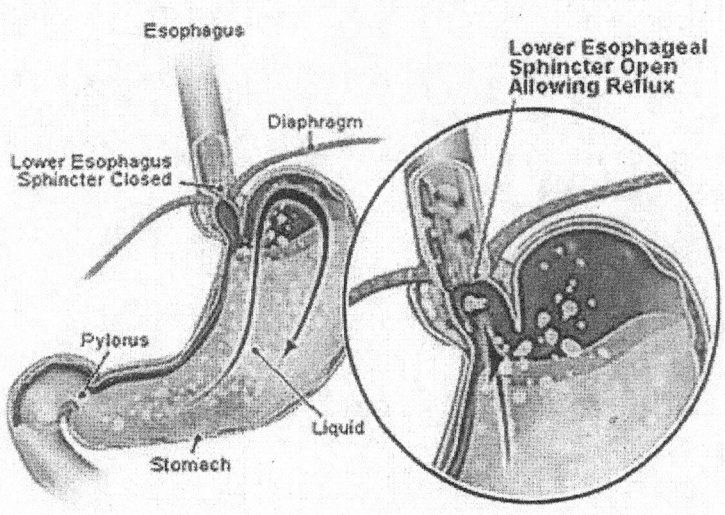

(Acidity Problem-Not to worry, 2010, www.caretips4u.blogspot.com)

The strong acidity of the stomach prevents bacterial growth and kills most bacteria that enter the body with food. It would destroy the cells of the stomach as well, but for their natural defenses. To protect themselves from gastric juice the goblet cells of the stomach wall secrete mucus, a thick, slippery, white substance that coats the cells, protecting them from the acid and enzymes that might otherwise harm them. The acidity of gastric juice registers below 2 on the pH scale- stronger than vinegar (Victoria, J etal, 2008).

But excessive acidity is most frequently due to the decomposition of the food and to a process of fermentation, dependent rather upon an insufficient amount of the gastric solvent than upon its superfluity. It then manifests itself after meals. When the

6

mucous membrane is covered with the tenacious mucous or with thick layers of epithelium, slow digestion and acidity from fermentation results; because, although the gastric juice is sufficient, it cannot mix as readily with the ailment.

The acids formed in the stomach are, besides the muriatic acid of the gastric juice, lactic acid, acetic acid, carbonic acid, butyric acid, and oxalic acid. Some articles of food produce these different acids in considerable quantities. Thus sugar generates large amount of lactic acid. The acids which are created in the stomach may get into the blood, and by vitiating that fluid give rise to various disorders.

When much acid is present in the viscus, it occasions a sensation of heat which extends along the esophagus; this condition is known as "heart burn".

Contributing factors of acid reflux/acidity

Dietary and life style choices may contribute to acid reflux by weakening the lower esophageal sphincter (LES). A weakened LES can make chronic reflux problems more likely. Those factors that may contribute to LES dysfunction and allow reflux are:

- Alcohol
- Chocolate
- Citrus fruits and juices
- Coffee
- Fried or fatty foods
- Nicotine
- Peppermint
- Some prescription medications

Avoiding these items can help prevent symptoms. In addition, certain conditions like pregnancy, obesity, hiatal hernias may predispose an individual to acid reflux distress according to many studies, and lying flat can make acid reflux symptoms worse, especially for individuals who lie down after a large meal (Gastroesophageal Reflux Disease, 2010, www.medicinenet.com).

- **Smoking**

Smoking is recognized as a major contributor to heartburn. Tobacco can reduce the production of saliva, which serve as a buffer for the lining of the esophagus. It may also cause the stomach to produce more acid, while relaxing the LES muscle between the stomach and the esophagus, making acid reflux more likely (Gastroesophageal Reflux Disease, 2010, www.medicinenet.com)..

- **Medications**

Some medications can also contribute to heartburn including over the counter drugs such as aspirin and ibuprofen (i.e. Advil, Motrin). Some drugs are less irritating if taken with food or milk (Gastroesophageal Reflux Disease, 2010, www.medicinenet.com).

- **Emptying of the stomach**

Most reflux during the day occurs after meals. This reflux probably is due to transient LES relaxations that are caused by distention of the stomach with food. The slower emptying of the stomach prolongs the distention of the stomach with food after meals. Therefore, the slower emptying prolongs the period of time during which reflux is more likely to occur (Gastroesophageal Reflux Disease, 2010, www.medicinenet.com).

- ## Hiatal hernias

Some doctors believe a hiatal hernia may also weaken the LES and cause acid reflux. Hiatal hernias occur when the upper part of the stomach moves up into the chest through a small opening in the diaphragm (diaphragmatic hiatus).

The diaphragm is the muscle separating the stomach from the chest. Recent studies show that the opening in the diaphragm acts as an additional sphincter around the lower end of the esophagus. These studies also reveal that hiatal hernias can also result in the retention of the acid and other contents above this opening, and these substances can reflux easily into the esophagus. Coughing, vomiting, straining or sudden physical exertion can cause increased pressure in the abdomen, which can lead to hiatal hernias. Obesity and pregnancy can also contribute to this condition. Many otherwise healthy people over age fifty have a small hiatal hernia. However, considered a condition of middle age, hiatal hernias affect the people of all ages (Kate Gilbert, U., 2001).

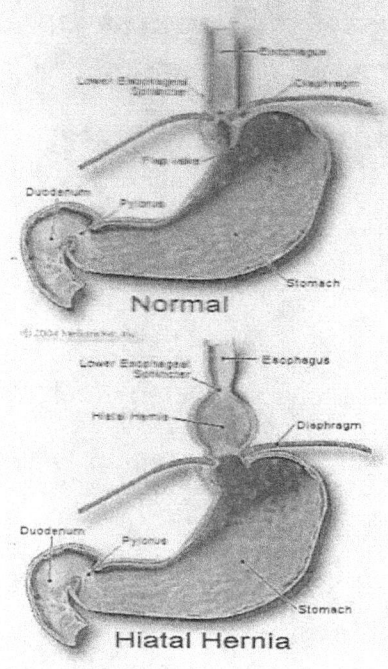

Normal

Hiatal Hernia

SYMPTOMS OF ACIDITY

- **Acid Regurgitation**

Regurgitation is the appearance of refluxed liquid in the mouth. In most patients with GERD, usually only small quantities of liquid reach the esophagus, and the liquid remains in the lower esophagus. Occasionally in some patients with GERD, larger quantities of liquid, sometimes containing food, are refluxed and reach the upper esophagus.

At the upper end of the esophagus is the upper esophageal sphincter (UES). The UES (upper esophageal sphincter) is a circular ring of muscle that is very similar in its actions to the LES (lower esophageal sphincter). That is, the UES prevents esophageal contents from backing up into the throat. When small amounts of refluxed liquid and/or foods breach (get through) the UES and enter the throat, there may be an acid taste in the mouth. If larger quantities reach the UES, patients may suddenly find their mouths filled with the liquid or food. What's more, frequent or prolonged regurgitation can lead to acid-induced erosions of the teeth (Gastroesophageal Reflux Disease, 2010, www.medicinenet.com).

- **Heart burn**

Heart burn is the painful sensation a person feels when the cardiac sphincter fails to prevent the stomach contents from refluxing into the esophagus (Victoria, J., 2008).

Food is passed through the esophagus into the stomach through a sphincter known as the lower esophageal sphincter (LES). That sphincter open and closes through a variety of involuntary muscular contractions known as peristalsis. For a number of reasons, the sphincter doesn't always completely shut after dumping ingested food particles into the stomach. So the food in the stomach acid comes back up the sphincter, causing a burning sensation in the chest and sometimes a spreading pain throughout the neck and arms that may even be mistaken for a heart attack. Person can also experience nausea, belching, and regurgitation of that half-digested food. When it comes back the sphincter, it doesn't taste as good as it did going down. This is clinically called acid reflux and in lay terms is known as heartburn or acid-indigestion. Heartburn/reflex usually lasts about two hours.

Symptoms of heartburn

There are a number of atypical or odd symptoms which include:

- Morning hoarseness

- Drooling

- Coughing spells

- Wake up with a sour throat

- Asthma like symptoms (or the worsening of asthma symptoms if one is asthmatic) (Rosenthal, S.M., 2001).

Heartburn discomfort starts behind the breast bone, rises to the chest and may extend to the neck, throat and face. Heartburn may be a sign of a more serious condition called gastro-esophageal reflux disease (GERD) (Mann, D., Feb 1999).

Causes

This may happen if a person eats or drinks too much (or both).people who overeat or eat too quickly are likely to suffer from indigestion. The muscular reaction of the stomach to un-chewed lumps or to being over-filled may be so violent that it causes regurgitation (reverse peristalsis). When this happens, over eaters may taste the stomach acid and feel pain. Back pressure from the stomach forces food up into the esophagus. Tight clothing and even changes of position (lying down, bending over) can cause it, too, as can some medications and smoking. A defect of the cardiac sphincter itself is a possible, but less likely cause (Victoria, J.etal., 2008).

Cures

If the heart burn is not caused by an anatomical defect, treatment is fairly simple. Tips for people suffering from heart burn include the following

1. Eat small meals.

2. Drink liquids one hour before or one hour after meal.

3. Refrain from lying down or bending over and from wearing tight fitting clothing, particularly after a meal.

4. Lose weight, if over-weight.

5. Elevate the head of the bed by 4-6 inches.

6. Avoid food, beverages and medicines that seem to aggravate the heartburn.

7. Refrain from smoking cigarettes.

8. Chewing gum may bring relief of symptoms by increasing the flow of saliva, which helps in re-swallowing the esophageal contents.

9. Use antacids infrequently for occasional heartburn, they may mask or cause problems, if used regularly (Rolfes, R. S etal, 2009).

CONDITIONS AFFECTING THE STOMACH

1. DYSPEPSIA

Dyspepsia (often called "indigestion") is the sensation of pain or discomfort in the upper abdomen that occurs after food consumption. Dyspepsia refers to the general symptoms of indigestion in the upper abdominal region, which may include stomach pain, gnawing sensations, early satiety, and nausea, vomiting and bloating. These symptoms sometimes indicate the presence of more serious illness, such as GERD (gastroesophageal reflux disease) or peptic ulcer disease (Rolfes, R. S etal, 2009).

Causes of dyspepsia

Abdominal symptoms don't always lead to a clear diagnosis, as the cause of the symptoms can be difficult to identify. Various medical conditions can cause abdominal discomfort; they include peptic ulcers, GERD, motility disorders, malabsorptive disorders, gall bladder disease, and tumors in the esophagus or stomach. Chronic disease such as diabetes mellitus, heart diseases and hypothyroidism can sometimes be accompanied by gastric symptoms. Some medications, including aspirin and other (nonsteroidal anti-inflammatory drugs), antibiotics, digitalis, and theophylline, can cause gastrointestinal distress. Dietary supplements may also be a cause; for example, iron and potassium supplements and some herbal products can cause gastrointestinal problems. Intestinal conditions such as irritable bowel syndrome or lactose intolerance may mimic dyspepsia. Although pinpointing the cause may be difficult, a complete examination is in order if the individual experiences weight loss, persistent vomiting, dysphagia, anemia, or bleeding, which suggest the presence of serious illness (Rolfes, R. S etal, 2009).

Potential food intolerances

Although many people attribute their symptoms to eating certain foods or spices, controlled studies have been unable to find associations between specific foods and dyspepsia. Coffee can induce symptoms in about 15 percent of dyspepsia patients, however, and also increases gastric acid production and acid reflux. Spicy foods may cause some injury to the mucosal lining and exacerbate the pain from a preexisting ulcer. High-fat-meals can slow gastric emptying and thereby exacerbate dyspepsia. To minimize symptoms, people with dyspepsia are sometimes advised to consume small meals with well cooked foods that are not overly seasoned and to consume meals in a relaxed atmosphere (Rolfes, R. S etal, 2009).

Bloating and stomach gas

The feeling of bloating may be caused by excessive gas in the stomach, which accumulates when air is swallowed. Swallowed air often accompanies gum chewing, smoking, rapid eating, drinking carbonated beverages, and using a straw. Omitting these practices generally helps to correct the problem (Rolfes, R. S etal, 2009).

2. FLATULANCE

Flatulence is the most common digestive disturbance. Most people have some gas; however, if the gas begins to cause discomfort, it may be an indication of a more complex problem (Kirschmann D. J., 2007).

The gas in the intestinal canal may be merely air that may be swallowed; or may be generated from imperfectly digested food; or it may be a secretion of the blood vessels from the part. In those who suffer from indigestion, it is produced in the last two ways, and the patient complains greatly of the annoyance it occasions. It causes disgust for eating, a feeling of distention, and sometimes actual pain. By interfering with the downward movements of the diaphragm, it induces a sensation of constriction in the chest, shortened breathing, and palpitation of the heart; and the sleep is broken by uneasy dreams (Kirschmann D. J., 2007).

An expulsion of the gaseous contents of the stomach by the mouth gives rise to eructation or belching. The belching that follows the decomposition of the food has sometimes the taste and odor of the rotten eggs, owing to the gas evolved, consisting of the sulphureted hydrogen. At other times, the eructation is odorless, because the gases formed are carbonic acid, or hydrogen or nitrogen or some of their compounds. When the gas results from fermentation or decomposition of food, it frequently coexists with acidity occurring only after meals. When it is a secretion from the blood vessels, it happens in the empty state of the stomach, and is often relieved by simply regulating the time of taking food, so as to avoid too long intervals between the meals (Kirschmann D. J., 1866).

3. GASTRITIS

Gastritis is a general term meaning "inflammation of the stomach" (19). Gastritis is a disease in which mucous lining of the stomach becomes irritated and inflamed. If gastritis is prolonged, the stomach walls become very thin and secretions are made up almost entirely of mucus, with very little digestive acid. In this condition, stomach is enable to produce intrinsic factor, a substance necessary for the absorption of vitamin B12, which the body needs for the formation of red blood cells. Thus the gastritis patients are in danger of developing pernicious anemia (Zand, J etal, 1999).

Symptoms

Gastritis can be painless even there is considerable disruption of the stomach lining (Zand, J., 1999).

Symptoms of gastritis include

- Indigestion (dyspepsia)
- Vomiting
- Headache
- Coated tongue

- Abnormal increase or decrease in appetite

- Diarrhea and abdominal cramps (DeBruyne, K. L etal, 2008).

Causes

The cause of gastritis appear to be

- Overindulgence in alcohol

- Smoking

- Coffee

- Highly seasoned or fried food (DeBruyne, K. L etal, 2008).

All these things increase the activity of stomach. Eating rancid food can cause bacterial infection, which may cause gastritis. Recurring causes of gastritis may be the result of peptic ulcer or of buildup of poisonous body wastes from such diseases as chronic uremia or cirrhosis of the liver. Any condition causing stress can bring on the symptoms of gastritis (DeBruyne, K. L etal, 2008).

Complications of gastritis

The extensive tissue damage that sometimes develops in chronic gastritis can disrupt gastric secretory function. If hydrochloric secretions become abnormally low (hypochlorhydria) or absent (achlorydria), absorption of nonheme iron and vitamin B12 can be impaired, and the risk of deficiencies increases. Pernicious anemia, a condition characterized by the destruction of stomach cells that produce intrinsic factor, is a late complication of atrophic gastritis and a primary cause of vitamin B12 deficiency (DeBruyne, K. L etal, 2008).

Another type of gastritis is "stress" gastritis, which occurs in surgical patients and people with serious medical problems, such as burns, trauma, massive infection, organ failure, cirrhosis of the liver, and acute local infections caused by a variety of bacteria, viruses, fungi, and even parasites. Exposure to radiation or caustic substances such as acids and drain cleaners can also cause this type of gastritis (Zand, J etal, 1999).

4. STOMACH ULCERS

Peptic ulcers are erosions that typically begin in the mucosal lining of the stomach and may penetrate into the deeper layers of stomach walls. They occur when the gastric mucosal barrier is disrupted, and thus pepsin and HCL acts on the stomach wall instead of the food in the lumen. Frequent backflow of the acidic gastric juices into the esophagus or excess or un-neutralized acid from the stomach in the duodenum can lead to peptic ulcers in these sites as well (Sherwood, L., 2010).

Pathogenesis

1. Helicobacter pylori

Helicobacter pylori contribute to the ulcer formation in part by secreting toxins that cause a persistent inflammation, or chronic superficial gastritis at the site it colonizes. H. pylori furthers weakens the gastric mucosal barrier by disrupting the tight junction between the gastric epithelial cells, thereby making the gastric mucosa leakier than normal (Sherwood, L., 2010).

Once the organism colonizes the human gastric mucosa, it induces inflammation and has the ability to persist for the life time in the individuals. The effect of the infection on gastric acid secretion is related to the distribution of the gastritis within the stomach, in particular to the extent to which it involves the antrum or the body of the stomach or both of these regions. The antral mucosa produces the hormone gastrin which circulates and stimulates the parietal cells in the body region of the stomach to secrete acid. In antrum predominant H.pylori gastritis, there is increased gastrin release and consequently increased acid secretion. This is the predominant gastritis seen in the patients with duodenal ulcer when both basal-and-meals stimulated acid outputs reported to be elevated (Sherwood, L., 2010).

2. NSAIDs

Alone or with conjunction with this infectious culprit, other factors are known to contribute to ulcer formation. Frequent exposure to some chemicals can break the gastric mucosal barrier, the most important of these are, ethyl alcohol and non-steroidal anti-inflammatory drugs (NSAID, s) such as aspirin, ibuprofen, or more potent medications, for the treatment of arthritis or other chronic inflammatory processes. Persistent stressful situations are frequently associated with ulcer formation, presumably because emotional stress can stimulate excessive gastric secretion.

When the gastric mucosal barrier is broken, acid and pepsin diffuse into the mucosa and underlying sub mucosa, with serious pathophysiological consequences. The surface erosion, or ulcer, progressively enlarges as increasing levels of acid, and pepsin continues to damage stomach wall. Two of the most serious consequences of ulcers are

1. Hemorrhage resulting from damage to sub mucosal capillaries and

2. Perforation, or complete erosion through the stomach wall, resulting in the escape of potent gastric contents into the abdominal cavity (Sherwood, L., 2010).

Effect of emotional stress

Although most ulcers result from either Helicobacter Pylori infection or NSAID use, an estimated 10 to 20 percent of ulcers develop in people who have no exposure to either. Emotional stress is not believed to cause ulcers per se, but it has effects on physiological processes and behaviors that may increase person vulnerability. Physiological effects of stress vary among individuals but may include rapid stomach emptying (which increase the acid load in the duodenum), hormonal changes that impair wound healing, and increases in acid and pepsin secretions. Stress may also lead to behavioral changes including increase use of alcohol, tobacco, and NSAIDs-all potential risk factors. Thus, stress may play a contributory role in ulcer development, although its precise effects are not fully understood (DeBruyne, K. L., 2008).

Signs and symptoms

Peptic ulcer symptoms vary. Some people are asymptomatic or experience only mild discomfort. Ulcer "pain" may be experienced as a hunger pain, a sensation of gnawing, or a burning pain in the stomach region. The pain or discomfort of ulcers may be relieved by food and recur several hours after a meal, especially if the ulcer is duodenal. Gastric ulcers may sometimes be aggravated by food and can cause loss of appetite and eventual weight loss. Ulcer symptoms tend to go into remission regularly and recur every few weeks or months (DeBruyne, K. L., 2008).

Complications of peptic ulcer

Peptic ulcers are a major source cause of gastrointestinal bleeding, which is the first sign of an ulcer in about 10 to 15 percent of cases. Bleeding is suspected if a person feels week or fatigued or shows other signs of anemia. Severe bleeding or hemorrhage is evidenced by black, tarry stools or, occasionally, vomit that resembles coffee grounds._Other serious complications of ulcer include perforations of the stomach or duodenum and gastric outlet obstruction (DeBruyne, K. L., 2008).

Drug therapies for ulcers

The goals of ulcer treatment are to relieve pain, promote healing, and prevent recurrence. Treatment often requires a combination of antibiotics to eradicate Helicobacter pylori infection and discontinuing the use of aspirin and other NSAIDs, which irritate the gastric mucosa and may delay healing. Antisecretory drugs may be prescribed to relieve pain and allow healing; these include proton-pump inhibitors, H2 blockers, or antacids (as used in GERD). Bismuth preparations (such as Pepto-Bismol) or sucralfate may help by coating the gastrointestinal lining and preventing further tissue erosion (DeBruyne, K. L., 2008)..

Dietary considerations

Alterations in diet are advised only if symptoms are affected by food consumption. As with gastritis, dietary recommendations are individualized to personal tolerances. The patients should avoid foods that may irritate the gastrointestinal lining such as alcohol, coffee, and caffeine containing beverages and spicy foods. Large meals should be avoided so that gastric secretions do not persist for long periods. There is no evidence that dietary supplements alter the rate of healing (DeBruyne, K. L., 2008).

Prevention

Recommendations for avoiding H. pylori infection involve washing hands thoroughly, eating foods that have been properly prepared, and drinking water from a clean source (Victoria, J_etal, 2008).

Treatment

The primary diagnostic technique used to examine the stomach lining is endoscopic examination-either gastroscopy, which is used to examine the stomach, or a procedure with the daunting name esophagogastroduodenoscopy (EGD), in which both the stomach and the duodenum, the first section of the small intestine, are examined. Either procedure involves inserting a flexible fiber-optic tube through the mouth and guiding it down the throat into (and possibly through) the stomach. The doctor can then looks directly at the stomach lining and determine the presence and extent of bleeding or eroded areas. This is not usually done, however, unless there is some question as to whether there is a more serious condition, such as an ulcer, or unless gastritis has become a chronic problem (Zand, J etal, 1999).

Conventional Treatment

- Over the counter antacids such as Mylanta, Maalox, or Rolaids are usually tried first. These agents have a short span of action, but with repeated use, they may inhibit stomach acid enough to disrupt digestion and interfere with the absorption of nutrients (Zand, J etal, 1999).

- A popular treatment (and preventive) is sucralfate (Carafate). This drug primarily used for ulcers farther down in the gastrointestinal tract, is used for gastritis because it seems to act as a protectant against acid, bile and pepsin. Possible side effects of this drug include constipation, and minor incidence of diarrhea, dry mouth, gas, itching, rash, and insomnia. Not much is absorbed into the blood stream but sucralfate does contain a significant amount of aluminum, which has been implicated as a possible cause of disease, and which has no known beneficial effect in the human body. Sucralfate can also interfere with the absorption of the many other types of drugs, including some antibiotics, epilepsy, medications, antifungal drugs, ulcer drugs, asthma drugs, and heart medications, so it should be taken separately from other drugs (Zand, J etal, 1999).

- Acid blockers may be used for variable lengths of time. Example includes cimetidine (Tagamet), famotidine (Pepcid), nizatidine (Axid), and ranitidine (Zantac). These drugs block acid secretion to lower stress on irritated stomach tissues. Possible side effects include constipation, diarrhea, nausea, vomiting, rash, occasional heart-rhythm changes, and blood-count changes. These drugs can pass into the breast milk, so nursing mothers should avoid them (Zand, J etal, 1999).

- A more recent type of medication used for gastritis is the proton pump inhibitor. Omeprazole (Prilosec) and lansoprazole (Prevacid) are two examples. These drugs also inhibit the production of stomach acid, but by a different mechanism than the one the acid blockers use. Possible side effects include headache, diarrhea, nausea, abdominal pain, pancreatic liver stress, and rashes.

- Avoid all nonsteroidal anti-inflammatories unless specifically directed to take them by doctors (Zand, J etal, 1999).

ANTACIDS

Drugs aimed at overcoming real or fancied over acidity are called gastric antacids. Their job is to neutralize excess hydrochloric acid and inactivate pepsin, two substances secreted by the stomach as a vital part of the digestive process (Pills and potions for indigestion, Feb 1974). Antacids are designed to help relieve the acute symptoms from abnormal conditions, such as the pain felt by an ulcer patient whose stomach or duodenal lining has been attacked by acid.

Antacids will provide quick relief, but they are not appropriate therapy for the stomach's discomfort. An antacid places a demand on the stomach to secrete more acid to counteract the neutralizer and enable the digestive enzymes to do their work. So the person still ends up with acid in the stomach, but the stomach has had to work against the antacid to produce it. So the person who over-eats or swallows un-chewed food needs to sit upright until the unhappy stomach has had a chance to cope with the problem it faces. Then to avoid such misery in the future the person needs to learn to eat less at a sitting, chew food more thoroughly and eat it more slowly (Whitney, N. E etal, 1996).

SOME MOST COMMON ANTACIDS

Antacids are not alike and none is ideal for every problem. Here's a description of the commonest antacids. Some types should be avoided by the people with kidney and heart problems (Pills and potions for indigestion, Feb 1974).

1. SODIUM BICARBONATE

Quickly neutralize Hydrochloric acid, providing quick relief from "acid indigestion". The effect however is brief. It generates carbon dioxide in the stomach, and because some salt formed by the chemical reaction is absorbed into the system, overdosing can aggravate a condition (alkalosis) that in the beginning produces same sort of symptoms that people take the drug to relieve (Pills and potions for indigestion, Feb 1974).

2. Calcium carbonate

Calcium carbonate is long lasting, quick acting and inexpensive. Used over long periods, it tends to constipate. Some drugs manufacturers combine it with, magnesium salt, a laxative, to overcome this (Pills and potions for indigestion, Feb 1974).

3. Aluminum hydroxide

It is slower acting than either of the forgoing and has the advantage of being safer for people with impaired kidney or circulatory functions who must limit their calcium intake. It is often combined with magnesium compounds to control constipation (Pills and potions for indigestion, Feb 1974).

4. Magnesium hydroxide

Magnesium hydroxide acts quickly, has good neutralizing ability and is relatively long lasting. The main ingredient is the same as milk of magnesia, a laxative, so it often comes as a preparation containing anti-diarrheals, such as calcium and aluminum.

Chronic takers with kidney impairment can build up dangerous levels of magnesium in their bodies (Pills and potions for indigestion, Feb 1974).

5. Magnesium trisillicate

It is a slower acting anti acid with long lasting activity. It has a relatively low neutralizing ability but has been shown effective in controlling ulcer pain.

People with heart problems also need to be on guard against certain antacids. Some are high enough in sodium to rule them out for the patients on low sodium diets.

Under a doctor's supervision, anti-acids are helpful in treating gastritis, peptic ulcers and hyperchlorydria, a condition in which stomach puts too much hydrochloric acid.

When anti acids relieve the pain of ulcers, there is no conclusive evidence that they make them heal any faster. The conditions likeliest to respond are "acid indigestion", "sour stomach" and "heartburn" a burning sensation in the center of the chest caused by stomach acid that is regurgitated into the esophagus (Pills and potions for indigestion, Feb 1974).

Incidentally, an antiacid taken after a meal continues working two to three hours, compared with about 15 minutes for one taken on an empty stomach (Pills and potions for indigestion, Feb 1974).

Dietary approach for acidity and related problems

Avoid fried food and highly seasoned foods. A low fat diet is necessary for those with a chronic condition. Frequent small meals are easier for the stomach to digest than fewer large meals. Acidic foods such as citrus, tomatoes, pineapple, and spicy foods can irritate a sore stomach. Alcohol, coffee, caffeinated sodas, carbonated drinks, aspirin, and other substances that irritate the stomach lining must be eliminated. Antacids may help (Kirschmann D. J., 2007).

An increase in alkalizing, no citrus juices, such as papaya, can be helpful. In addition, fresh papaya contains the enzyme papain that helps in digesting proteins, and some starches, and can also guard against the development of ulcers caused by taking large doses of aspirin. Other recommended foods are brown rice, pasta, potatoes and yogurt with active-culture acidophilus. Whole grains are preferred to refined white flour of cakes and cookies because whole grains trigger a slower secretion of gastric acid and contain protein, which help neutralize this acid. Chewing food thoroughly and relaxing when eating meals will do wonders for the stomach.

Nutrients may be beneficial. If gastritis is severe, iron supplements and injections of vitamin B12 may be helpful for preventing pernicious anemia. Herbs that may be helpful are goldenseal infusion and white willow as a substitute for aspirin with none of the side effects to the stomach (pregnant women do not take this herb). Exercise is very good for the stomach; any kind of enjoyable activity is recommended (Kirschmann D. J., 2007).

Pantothenic acid has been shown to relieve intestinal gas and distention where there is no physical cause. Gas pains were relieved in postoperative patients and prevented in others, when they were given 250 milligrams of pantothenic acid daily. Pantothenic acids aids in bowel motility and efficient digestion. Without pantothenic acid, acetylcholine can not be produced. This chemical transmits messages to nerves that control the motor and secretory activities of the intestine. Charcoal tablets are relief for gas (Kirschmann D. J., 2007).

. Fermented foods such as yogurt and buttermilk aid in the digestion of high-fiber and other foods by increasing friendly bacteria in the colon. They are also well tolerated by people who have lactase deficiency. Other foods that may be helpful are lemon juice and cider vinegar. Soy-sauce, cheese and alcohol should be avoided. Carbonated drinks only add more air. To counter the effects of some foods, there are natural products on the market that neutralize flatulence.

Carminative herbs stimulate digestion, by increasing gastric juices, decreasing the amount of putrefactive bacteria, and stimulating intestinal motility. These include garlic, magnolia bark, sweet flag infusion, fennel, ginger infusion, orange or lemon peel, and caraway. In traditional cuisines, found in various countries, certain classic dishes include herbs considered to reduce gas. For instance, in Mexican cooking, beans are cooked with the native herb epazote. Exercise stimulates intestinal peristalsis and helps break down large gas bubbles (Kirschmann. D. J., 2007).

REFRENCES

1. Acidity Problem-Not to worry (Tuesday, June 29, 2010). Retrieved August 28 2010, from http://caretips4u.blogspot.com/2010/06/acidity-problem-not-to-worry.html

2. DeBruyne, K. L, Pinna, K and Whitney Noss, E. (2008). Nutrition and diet therapy, 7th edition.USA: Thomson Learning.

3. Gastroesophageal Reflux Disease (GERD). (September 7, 2010). Retrieved 15 May,2010, from http://www.medicinenet.com/gastroesophageal_reflux_disease_gerd/page3.htm.

4. Guyton, A. C and John E. H (2006). Textbook of Medical Physiology, 11 edition: Philadelphia: Elsevier Saunders. p. 797.

5. Retrieved 21 July, 2010, from http://eatwellgetwell.files.wordpress.com/2006/05/digestion_good2.jpg

6. Kate Gilbert, U . (2001). Managing Acid Reflux, USA: Woodland publishers.

7. Kirschmann, D. J. (1866). Medical diagnosis with special reference to practical medicine, 2nd edition: J.B Lippincott &CO.

8. Kirschmann D. J.(2007). Nutrition Almanac, 6TH EDITION. USA: McGraw Hill companies.

9. Mann, D. (Feb 1999). Health in balance (Better Nutrition): Primedia Enthusiastic Publications.

10. Minocha, A and Carroll, D. (2003).   Natural stomach care. USA: Penguin group

11. Pills and potions for indigestion. (Feb 1974). Kiplinger's Personal Finance (Changing times). USA: Austin H. Kiplinger.

12. Rosenthal, S.M.(2001). 50 ways to relieve heartburn, reflux, and ulcers. USA: R.R. Donnelley and sons.

13. Rolfes, R. S. Pinna, K and Whitney, E. (2009). Understanding normal and clinical nutrition, 8th edition. Canada: Yolanda Cossio

14. Sherwood, L. (2010). Human Physiology: from cells to systems, 7th edition. USA: Yolanda Cossio.

15. Stomach acidity symptoms, Reduce stomach acid naturally, Stomach acid diet (28 july 2008). Retrieved August 26 2010, from http://www.home-remedies-for-you.com/askquestion/18844/stomach-acidity-symptoms-reduce-stomach-acid-natur.html

16. Stomach acidity – one of the most widespread humanity disease (21 Sep 2007). Retrieved August 10 2010, from http://stomachacidity.com/

17. Victoria, J and Fraser, M.d. (2008). Diseases and disorders. Malaysia: Paul Bernabeo.

18. Whitney, N. E and Rolfes, R.S. (1996). Understanding nutrition, 7th edition. New York: West publishing company.

19. Zand, J. Allan N. Spreen, James B. LaValle. (1999). Smart Medicine for Healthier Living. USA: Avery publishing group.